TABLE OF CONTENTS

BIG FAT DISCLAIMER:

While every effort has been made to accurately represent how to avoid hangovers without giving up your favorite booze, there is no guarantee you will prevent hangovers. Any product that tells you otherwise is lying. Even though the strategy laid out for you, within this eBook, is the best possible way to prevent hangovers, there is never any guarantee.

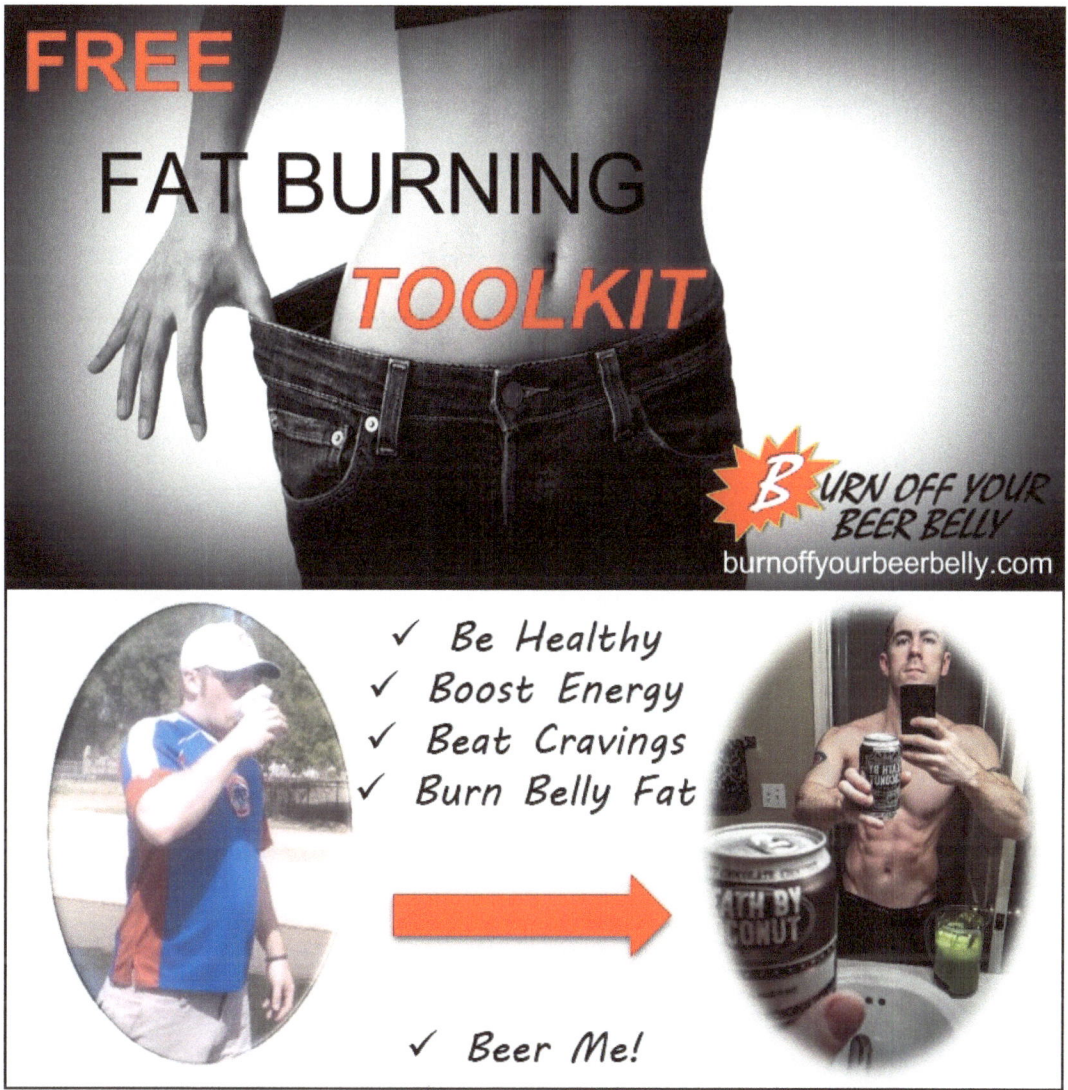

FREE FAT BURNING TOOLKIT - get all the Free tools I used to lose 54lbs, boost energy, beat cravings, prevent hangovers and burn off my beer belly:

http://www.burnoffyourbeerbelly.com/toolkit

52 HANGOVER-FREE WEEKENDS

Never Give Up Your Favorite Booze

The Ultimate Guide To Hangover Prevention

By Ryan Jerome

INTRODUCTION

My Story And Why You Should Read This Book

"I'm never drinking again!", I groaned from underneath my cave of bed covers, early afternoon on January 1st, 2011. This was only, I'd say, the 832,496th time I had spewed these words to the heavens. Never once had I actually followed through with this ludicrous statement, but maybe this time…

Umm, that's a negative…

But, it was about that time I started thinking maybe I should make some real changes to my lifestyle. I was tired of waking up to horrendously violent hangovers on the weekends.

Although, the night before was always so much fun - I didn't want to give up the fun, I only wanted to give up the hangovers.

Was this even possible? Is there a way to design my lifestyle so that I could avoid hangovers without giving up my favorite booze? A way to biohack my body & mind to create incredible health and wellness while still enjoying my sinful craft beers & microbrews?

I made it my mission to create a yearly lifestyle of 52 hangover-free weekends without giving up my favorite booze. Now, I want to share what I found with you.

We, that enjoy our favorite booze, need to stick together. Our *'morning-afters'* are getting tougher to handle. Not to mention, the horrible toll it's taking on our bodies.

The good news? Once you understand the whole process and these proven strategies, it actually becomes quite simple to prevent hangovers, every single time.

Some of what I share with you may seem weird, unconventional and downright ludicrous. I expect you to have those feelings, to be skeptical of the hangover prevention methods I use every weekend.

Don't let those feelings keep you from testing everything yourself. You have already purchased this eBook, why not give it a try?

I'm confident you'll benefit greatly from implementing all the simple techniques discussed within this book.

It's your party, live it healthy & hangover-free!

ABOUT THE AUTHOR

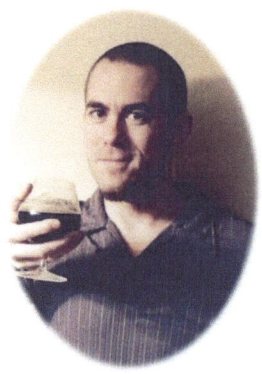

Before becoming a hangover-free, craft beer drinking, body fat burning author, Ryan Jerome was an overweight, beer drinking, cubicle dwelling, unproductive, unhealthy mess. Truly a hot mess!

Queue the 2011 mindset shift. The new awakening. An educational journey of mind expansion, productivity, efficiency and rejection of mainstream wisdom. He dared to be unconventional.

Ryan started blogging at avoidinghangovers.com, but has since shifted more of his attention over to burnoffyourbeerbelly.com. There, he's helping booze drinkers be healthy, boost energy, beat cravings, banish hangovers and burn off their beer bellies!

He has Freely detailed how he effectively lost 54lbs, increased productivity, boosted energy levels, destroyed cravings, expanded cognitive function, built lean muscle, prevented hangovers and ultimately burned off his own beer belly without giving up his favorite craft beers.

Here's what health and fitness trainer Jay Cardiello said about Ryan Jerome:

"Ryan, you're doing a wonderful job and being very informative. What you're introducing, to a lot of people, is a celebration of life. We all don't do it enough, celebrate your healthy life!"

- Jay Cardiello from the No-Diet Plan on ABC TV's My Diet Is Better Than Yours, jcardio.com

Here's what other booze drinkers are saying about Ryan Jerome:

"YEAH Ryan! I love your philosophy. This info of yours has been most valuable because it is so unconventional. You've helped me avoid hangovers and all the ills of drinking. Knowledge is power, my friend. Thank you for speaking the truth."

- Roger

"Thank you, this was the scientific approach to hangovers, I was looking for!"

- Garth

"Thanks, Ryan Jerome, for this useful eBook to keep me hangover free."

- Sarah

"You've provided exactly the kind of answer I was looking for to cure my hangovers for good."

- Craig

"I really appreciate the time you have taken to clearly advise me on burning body fat and avoiding hangovers, Ryan. This is exactly the advice I've been seeking. Your hangover cures can easily be a 'break through' if you will... I know that word sounds a bit 'markety' but if marketed well, could really help many, many people out there. I cannot tell you how grateful I am, and how much appreciation I feel after receiving your advice."

- Kabir

"You have taken out so much time, to write to someone you have never met before – hats off to your kind selflessness. Also, the replies in themselves have given me much needed clarity. I am the kind of person who needs to go right down to the bottom of things before my mind fully accepts, and has conviction about whatever it is – only then I am propelled to act with more decisiveness, surety and clarity. Thank you. Thank you. Thank you."

- Kabir (again)

"Hey Ryan! Thank you so much for taking the time to provide me with a plan to try out, it's really working wonderfully. I've found that when I start my morning with foods that are more dense and less sugary, my tendency to snack during the day lessens. I had one semi busy day where I almost worked right through lunch, where my stomach usually tells me it's time to go. I also feel a greater boost of energy, less sluggish and more empowered to do my workouts every night. Thanks again!"

- Rachel :)

"Ryan, from Burn Off Your Beer Belly, has helped me stay energized and focused all day without craving all the extra junk our bodies don't need. I'm losing weight and feeling great! Thank you!"

- Jefe

"I'm very excited to start eating healthier and lose my belly fat! The mouthwatering recipes are awesome. I really like the personalized suggestions and tips from Ryan Jerome to help keep me on track! Thanks for giving me the guidance I need!"

- Sharon

"Thanks so much Burn Off Your Beer Belly! I've been losing 5 or 6 pounds a week, since following your advice. I love your podcast and website, they are excellent resources. Keep them coming!"

- Roger

Hey Ryan! I just discovered your podcast and I love it. Thanks and keep burning!

- Stephen

YOU WILL DISCOVER…

- ✓ What the alcohol breakdown process is, within your body that leads to hangovers.
- ✓ How to hack this process with a powerful pre-drinking requisite that will prepare your body to fight off hangovers.
- ✓ A couple drink recipes that will boost your body's immune system before you start tipping back the booze.
- ✓ A very potent supplement protocol to help promote your liver's detoxifying process.
- ✓ What the most effective hangover prevention foods are to eat before, during and after drinking.
- ✓ Alcoholic drinks that are least likely to give you a hangover.
- ✓ An essential post-drinking requisite to follow before passing out.
- ✓ And the most practical *'morning after'* hangover cures that actually work.

What will you do with your new-found health, wellness, energy, productivity, vibrance and refreshing attitude during your 52 hangover-free weekends?

The possibilities are endless and exciting to think about.

Cheers to YOU! Let's jump in...

THE PROCESS

Hangovers Are Like Spam Email

Throughout my college days and most of my 20s the extent of my knowledge about hangovers was that, if I partied too hard, I would feel like shit the next day. Sure, everybody always said to eat greasy food and drink plenty of water - stay hydrated!

Or even drink Gatorade the next morning to replenish those electrolytes.

But, why was this passed around as the Holy Grail for dealing with hangovers? It never seemed to actually work for me. I even ditched the Gatorade for a baby sickness drink - Pedialyte. This still provided no real relief.

As I aged, it seemed like my weekend hangovers were getting worse. All these supposed hangover cures were not working. If I partied too hard Saturday night, Sunday was absolutely destroyed for me… I would still have lingering symptoms even on Monday! "What is happening!?!?"

I didn't know it at the time but that was the ultimate question, *what is happening?* If I seriously wanted to prevent hangovers without giving up my favorite booze, I needed to understand the process taking place inside my body while I was drinking.

After that infamous New Year's Day of 2011, I decided to learn all that I could about this process, in hopes that I could start cheating on hangovers. I'm no scientist or great thinker, but I do enjoy trying to figure out simplified hacks, so I don't have to deal with un-enjoyable activities. Take email as a real world example.

Almost everyone uses a simplified hack to help you handle spam emails. Your email provider will flag them as spam so they are dropped into a completely different folder, or you can set up **your own rules** to flag emails you never want to see, as spam. Think of email as social drinking and spam email as hangovers.

I wanted to set up **the ultimate rule** to flag hangovers as spam, so I never had to deal with them again. All while still enjoying social drinking.

The Hangover Process That Keeps Punching You In The Liver

This is no secret I've uncovered, you can find this process all over the internet and/or from legit doctors. But, as I mentioned earlier, I like things simplified. I'm no doctor, nor am I interested in becoming one.

Here is a simplified non-doctor, non-scientist analysis of the hangover process.

Almost immediately after you start consuming alcohol, your body *(specifically your liver)* starts metabolizing it. An enzyme called dehydrogenase, present in your body, begins to breakdown the alcohol. This alcohol breakdown process leads to the creation of a chemical called, acetaldehyde.

I'd like to introduce you to your hangover culprit, acetaldehyde. It is more toxic and harmful to your body than the alcohol itself.

Not only does it cause hangovers, but it's what gives you a lot of the other ill feeling effects, you may experience when drinking alcohol. Rapid pulse, nausea, vomiting, flushed skin, sweating, muscle fatigue, headache, etc...

While there are other aspects of drinking alcohol that can lead to a hangover, like toxic congeners, gut inflammation, or the frequent urination that depletes the body of other essential vitamins & minerals, **acetaldehyde should still be your main concern.**

We'll cover the other causes later in this book. But for now, how do we get rid of acetaldehyde?

Great question! That was my question, once I finally understood the hangover process. The answer is easier than you may think.

Your body already does it.

It's part of your natural detox process. There is a VERY powerful antioxidant, called glutathione, present throughout your whole body. Glutathione **attacks and destroys** acetaldehyde - *praise thee, oh magnificent one!*

So, if glutathione is present throughout your body and it attacks all the acetaldehyde, then why do you still get hangovers when drinking alcohol!?!?

The problem is, that you keep drinking more and more. Your body **only produces so much glutathione** and has a limited amount stored up.

With increasing amounts of acetaldehyde building up, you are **quickly and severely** depleting all of your body's glutathione. There's not enough glutathione present or being produced quick enough to effectively fight off the acetaldehyde.

You either quit drinking after a couple or you end up with a hangover the morning after.

Are you satisfied with that answer?

Or does it get you asking more questions?

The big question I had was:

HOW DO I INCREASE MY BODY'S GLUTATHIONE LEVELS BEFORE DRINKING?

I'm pretty sure that's what you were thinking too.

PRE-DRINKING REQUISITE

Boost That Glutathione

Wide-eyed with a new sense of intrigue, it was time to do some research experiments and self-studies. If I could figure out how to increase my body's glutathione levels, I could rule the world! *(Insert evil laugh... MUHAHAHA!)*

Okay, so maybe I couldn't rule the world - but I would definitely have way more control over myself, particularly, my insides. Since acetaldehyde is the biggest cause of hangovers, I would be well on my way to creating those 52 hangover-free weekends I've been yearning for.

Aren't you happy that I've already done all this research for you? Now it's time to simplify it! Buckle up, crack open that beer, pop that cork, pour that stiff one and follow along closely.

Here is a list of foods, vitamins and supplements, I've discovered, that all help to boost your body's glutathione levels *(I'll cover each one in more detail)*:

- N-Acetyl Cysteine *(aka NAC)*
- Alpha Lipoic Acid *(aka ALA)*
- Non-Denatured Native Whey Protein
- Cruciferous Vegetables
- Vitamin B Complex
- Liposomal Glutathione
- Liposomal Vitamin C
- Milk Thistle
- Grass-Fed Beef Liver
- Selenium

N-Acetyl Cysteine (NAC)

This has become my *'go-to'* supplement for powerful, yet cheap hangover prevention. NAC not only powers up your body's glutathione levels, it also binds acetaldehyde itself, thus preventing those damaging effects. It has proven to be so beneficial that I've added it to my daily supplement requisite whether I happen to be drinking or not.

Take at least one NOW Foods 600mg NAC capsule **before** consuming alcohol.

Alpha Lipoic Acid (ALA)

If you're not familiar with the supplement game, I can only imagine what you're thinking about these crazy names. Some of them sound like they could be forms of black market drugs. I assure you they aren't, you can buy these supplements from Amazon or at your local vitamin store.

ALA, like glutathione, is one of the most important antioxidants in your body. This means it protects cells and DNA from damage by free radicals and other toxins.

It also helps to increase your body's glutathione levels. While you're tipping back your favorite booze, you're going to need all the glutathione you can get - ALA will help you do just that.

Take at least one Doctor's Best 600mg ALA capsule before consuming alcohol.

Non-Denatured Native Whey Protein

That's a mouthful...

The best formulation to receive glutathione boosting proteins is cow's milk whey protein in undenatured form. What does undenatured mean? It's basically raw cow's milk - non pasteurized, non-homogenized - whey protein.

As always, look to make sure the cows are grass-fed. The group of proteins within whey, contain a large amount of cysteine - which leads to increased levels of glutathione.

Drink a Wild Whey Protein shake before consuming alcohol.

Cruciferous Vegetables

There has been several scientific studies done showing that the addition of cruciferous vegetables to your diet has a direct effect on your body's glutathione levels. The vegetables that increase those levels the most are broccoli, cabbage, brussels sprouts, kale, cauliflower and mustard.

At Burn Off Your Beer Belly, we always recommend eating broccoli with Kerrygold grass-fed butter melted all over them, before consuming alcohol.

Vitamin B Complex

While all B vitamins help to keep hangovers away, the top of the line is B1. Vitamin B doesn't necessarily increase your body's glutathione levels but it provides the same desired effect.

Let me explain…

Vitamin B1 deficiency can lead to things like fatigue, impaired awareness, loss of equilibrium, disorientation, memory loss, and muscle weakness. Alcohol consumption will deplete your Vitamin B1 levels and produce those exact same effects.

By boosting your Vitamin B levels, before consuming alcohol, you will decrease these effects - in the same way that increased glutathione levels decreases all those effects.

Take at least one NOW Foods 100mg Vitamin B1 before consuming alcohol.

Grass-Fed Beef Liver

Eat some liver and onions before you drink… I'm serious! Your body's glutathione levels will spike so much after eating Grass-Fed Beef Liver. It contains all the precursor amino acids needed, along with something called Hepatocyte Growth Factor (HGF) - *also known as liver cell growth factor.*

A research group recently had these findings…

"HGF turns on routes to produce natural antioxidant compounds in our body, for example a small tripeptide called glutathione which works as a very important antioxidant and liver protector."

"We have seen in this laboratory that ***HGF notably increases the production of glutathione and other protector compounds, not just for the liver, but for all the organs in the body: lungs, kidneys, pancreas, etc.*** *When this natural antioxidant is induced to increase its production, it protects the body from the toxic effects of many compounds like alcohols."*

Do yourself a solid, and have Tendergrass Farms or US Wellness Meats deliver grass-fed beef liver right to your door.

Selenium

If you enjoy the booze, most likely you have a deficiency in Selenium. Just so you know, having low levels of Selenium in your body can increase the risks of colon and liver cancer.

I don't mean to be a Debbie-Downer, but it's true. Don't worry, this is why I wrote the book - I want to help you stay healthy and hangover-free.

Let's reduce those risks by a huge margin by supplementing with Selenium. You'll keep your body healthy and boost those glutathione levels at the same time.

Don't overdo this, only take one NOW Foods 200mcg *(that's micrograms!)* Selenium capsule before consuming alcohol.

Liposomal Glutathione

Much more expensive than NAC, but a far more effective way to increase your glutathione levels is Liposomal Glutathione. I can't justify taking this every day since the cost can add up, but I most definitely add it to my pre-drinking requisite.

If you do incorporate a glutathione supplement to your requisite, please make sure it is Liposomal. The problem with a *'regular'* glutathione supplement is that your stomach enzymes will digest it before your gut is able to absorb it and deliver it to your liver, through your blood.

Liposomes are able to cross this barrier allowing for better absorption and protection.

Mix in at least 2 teaspoons of Vida Lifescience Mega Liposomal Glutathione into our featured drink recipes.

Liposomal Vitamin C

Studies have proven that taking in more Vitamin C will increase the glutathione levels in your body. While you could take a couple Vitamin C capsules, you'll run into the same kind of problem as with a *'regular'* glutathione capsule - only not as hardcore.

Your body may not absorb ANY of the *'regular'* glutathione capsule, while absorption rates can vary with Vitamin C capsules - usually in the 60 - 80% range. Get nearly 100% absorption rate by taking Liposomal Vitamin C & Liposomal Glutathione!

Mix in at least 2 teaspoons of [Vida Lifescience Liposomal Vitamin C](#) into our featured drink recipes.

Milk Thistle Extract

This little flower does so much more than look beautiful. Milk Thistle is another powerful antioxidant. It protects from DNA damage, especially in the liver and helps to increase glutathione levels.

There is clinical evidence showing Milk Thistle Extract as a treatment for alcohol-induced cirrhosis of the liver and other alcohol-induced liver diseases. Why the hell wouldn't you take this supplement before boozin' it up?!

Mix in a few drops of Botanic Choice Milk Thistle Extract into our featured drink recipes.

HANGOVER PREVENTION DRINK RECIPES

Green Detox Juice

[Grab your juicer here...](#)

Run these foods through your juicer:

- Cucumber
- Apple
- Lemon
- Turmeric Root
- Ginger Root
- Celery
- Kale

Next, stir these things into your juice:

- Liposomal glutathione
- Liposomal vitamin C
- Milk thistle extract
- Turmeric powder
- Black pepper
- Liquid fish oil

Or take the easier route with the **Detox Lemon Water**

- Large glass of water
- Half a lemon
- Liposomal glutathione
- Liposomal vitamin C
- Milk thistle extract
- Teaspoon of pink Himalayan sea salt

PROTECT AGAINST ALCOHOL INFLAMMATION

Another big contributor to those awful hangovers is inflammation from drinking alcohol. This alcohol inflammation can lead to more serious side-effects including alcohol related diseases.

Do I have your attention now?

The good news is there are legitimate ways to reduce and protect against alcohol inflammation before you start sipping on your favorite booze.

By increasing your body's glutathione levels, as previously mentioned, you've already thrown up a more serious line of defense against hangovers and alcohol inflammation than most people.

But, many people have differing types of inflammatory responses to drinking alcohol. Because of this, you should take every precaution available to you.

If you start drinking with dinner, make sure you're eating the correct foods. Yes, there are foods that protect your body from alcohol inflammation!

Make sure you're eating some or all of these foods for dinner and later that night if you get the drunken munchies.

Here's a simple checklist to help you out.

- ✓ Grass-Fed Meat
- ✓ Turmeric
- ✓ Avocados & Bananas
- ✓ Vegetables
- ✓ Grass-Fed Butter
- ✓ Pastured Eggs
- ✓ Nuts

Now think back to the last time you drank alcohol. Did you eat any of these 7 foods before or during your alcohol consumption?

Let's talk about how each of these foods can protect against alcohol inflammation.

WARNING This might make you very hungry...

Grass-Fed Beef

Typically, any type of meat will do, beef is always more readily available and cheaper than other types of meat. The most important part is that it's grass-fed, you won't be getting your omega-3 essential fatty acids and vitamin K2 by eating corn or grain fed meat.

Omega3s directly reduce inflammation and vitamin K2 protects your brain. Why wouldn't you eat grass-fed beef before drinking alcohol?

If you make grass-fed burgers, do not eat them on a bun. Carbohydrate loading, before drinking, to keep hangovers away is a big fat myth.

Instead, you want to load up on healthy fats. So, throw the burgers on a spinach or kale wrap, or better yet, treat yourself to a nice cut of grass-fed steak.

And cook everything in grass-fed butter!

Turmeric

The previously mentioned grass-fed steak should be well-seasoned with this stuff.

The best way to consume it is by juicing with the root – it's a lot like ginger root in that sense. And, always plays a major role in my pre-drinking green detox juice.

One of the active ingredients in turmeric root is curcumin which has a huge range of beneficial effects on the body – Anti-inflammatory, antibacterial, antiviral, antioxidant and glutathione booster.

It also increases the flow of bile, in the liver, soothing the stomach and balancing upset digestion from drinking alcohol – it's even been known to reduce alcohol-related ulcers.

This may very well be the most important spice in your rack or cabinet. Go ahead and SUPER-charge your body's absorption of this amazing little spice by mixing in some black pepper.

Avocados & Bananas

If you aren't eating avocados on a daily basis, you are harming not only your taste buds, but a lot of key components inside your body. Avocados are rich in potassium, like bananas, but – in my opinion – taste far superior.

Necessary potassium for proper nerve and muscle function is quickly depleted and expelled from your body through the urine when you're drinking alcohol.

Along with helping the body to replenish this potassium, avocados are also a strong antioxidant that can calm upset stomachs and headaches – as well as BOOST your glutathione levels and decrease inflammation.

These make a great drinking snack, too.

Vegetables

As was mentioned earlier for their glutathione boosting abilities, since they're high in cysteine.

Cysteine is a crucial amino acid and an essential organic compound that promotes the production & storage of glutathione.

They also reduce inflammation. I highly recommend cooking them in grass-fed butter for even more inflammation protection.

Grass-Fed Butter

Butter from grass-fed cows isn't like any other butter you've had. This type of butter is LOADED with essential omega-3 fatty acids to protect your body from inflammation. It really helps that it also tastes amazing!

My favorite brand is Kerrygold. You can even buy it in bulk and freeze it for future consumption.

It's also high in vitamin K2 to help protect that brain of yours.

Pastured Eggs

Eggs are a good source of omega-3 fatty acids, cysteine and vitamin B. You want to try and find organic, pastured eggs from cage-free hens as they tend to be of better quality.

The best way to get all the incredible benefits from eggs is to consume them raw, your body will absorb even more of the cysteine – this will boost your glutathione levels even higher.

But, if you're like me and eating raw eggs doesn't appeal to you, go ahead and fry an egg and toss it on your grass-fed burger! Or go sunny side up! You'll still reap plenty of the hangover prevention benefits.

Nuts

While cashews or pecans are good nuts to eat to help in hangover prevention, the best nuts are almonds.

Almonds are high in vitamin E, fats and oils that support liver function.

They also contain blood sugar balancing proteins. If you're going to eat any nuts before your night out partying or as a drinking snack, go for raw almonds.

DRINKING ALCOHOL TO NOT GET A HANGOVER

Beer Is Not The Best

Sadly, it's very true.

I love drinking delicious craft beers and micro brews. There's such a vast selection, my Untappd numbers rise every week. But, the best alcoholic drink for avoiding hangovers is not beer.

Although, craft beers and micro brews tend to be of a better quality and have fewer congeners than those typical, corporate mass-produced piss water beers.

It all comes down to a funny little word... congeners.

Congeners are hangover-inducing substances that are produced during the fermentation of alcohol. They're also produced in the liver during the breaking down of alcohol. We've discussed the biggest congener, acetaldehyde, earlier.

But, there are many more of these horrible congeners.

Chemicals like acetone, esters, tannins and aldehydes. These guys are responsible for most of the taste and aroma of your alcoholic beverages.

On one side, your favorite sweet, red wine tastes so good, because of these bad guy congeners but on the other side you're going to experience wicked hangovers because of them.

Try To Stay Away From Darker Drinks

Different types of alcohol contain different amounts & types of these nasty congeners. This is why you should stick to one type of alcohol all night. This will allow your liver to work on breaking down only the congeners included with that one type of alcohol.

Beer, along with other darker alcohols – like red wines, tequila and whiskey – contain more congeners than clearer alcohols do.

With the greater presence of congeners in darker alcohols, that leaves us with the clear stuff as the best alcohol to drink.

Drinking Clear = No Hangover Fear

TOP 3 ALCOHOLS TO STAY HANGOVER-FREE

Vodka

This is the #1 least likely alcoholic drink to cause a hangover. This does NOT mean you can go out for your night of drinking and down a whole fifth of it – then expect to wake up feeling fine in the morning. Vodka tends to be higher in alcohol – so as always - in moderation!

I recommend going for the potato vodka over the grain vodka if you have the choice. Also, if you're mixing something with your vodka, keep it water based – Tonic Water, Club Soda or even San Pellegrino Mineral Water is best.

Gin

Definitely the second least likely to cause a hangover. Gin is closely related to vodka as they are both grain alcohols *(unless you get the previously recommended potato vodka)*. The difference with gin is that it is flavored with juniper and isn't filtered as much as vodka.

You may want to try a natural, organic juice that is jam packed with vitamin C to mix with – as the vitamin C will help boost those glutathione levels and fight against a hangover – or just go with some San Pellegrino.

Clear Rum

All the clearer alcohols have fewer toxic congeners in them. If you're going with Rum for the night, dodge the dark rum and mix it with San Pellegrino.

The reason rum falls behind vodka and gin is because rum is made from sugar cane derivatives like fermented fresh cane juice or molasses. Sugar contributes, somewhat, to the severity of a hangover – but clear rum is still a better choice than dark rum or other dark alcohols.

POST DRINKING REQUISITE

I'm Finished Drinking, Can I Pass Out Now?

No, please don't! You need to stay awake a little longer. There are still a few simple things you need to do to make sure you've made it impossible for a hangover to arise in the morning.

Whenever I'm done drinking for the night, I always seem to be quite hungry. I assume the same happens to most people.

What do you usually do when this happens? Eat some leftover shit food? Maybe you hit up some fast-food joint on the way home? These are horrible ways to protect yourself from a hangover.

If you've got time and don't mind putting in the effort, you could cook yourself a nice grass-fed steak… seasoned with turmeric powder and black pepper.

For most people that's not a realistic option. They just want to shovel some food in so they can go pass out. No problem, why not grab an avocado? Avocados are my go-to after-drinking, before-bed, food.

Of course, you also want to drink plenty of water. Hydrate! You should have drank plenty of water during the course of your night as well. Many so-called experts claim that you need to drink one glass or bottle of water for every one alcoholic drink you consume.

I call BS on that. Sure, you definitely need to drink some water but you can make things a lot worse for your body if you over-do it. Be conscious of how much water you're drinking throughout the night and keep it *'in moderation'*.

The last thing you should do before passing out, and it may be the most important, is to take a couple activated charcoal capsules. This will aid in your body's detoxing process while you're sleeping.

It's more than likely, if you drank alcohol all night, that some of the nasty congeners specifically acetaldehyde have slipped through your **glutathione defense**. You must take care of these toxins before the next morning.

It's time for a little helpful clean up.

Activated charcoal capsules are your last line of defense against the hangover. These capsules are created by burning sources of carbon, like wood or coconut shells. The burning removes all the oxygen and activates it with steam & other gases which produces an extremely high absorbing material.

This material is packed with millions of tiny pores that can suck up and remove toxins, heavy metals, chemicals or other poisons that have thousands of times more weight than the charcoal itself. **It's really pretty incredible.**

Take them.

Now you may pass out, and while it may not be easy, you should try and get 7 - 9 hours of quality deep sleep.

THE MORNING AFTER

If you followed everything we've discussed, then you should wake up feeling refreshed and ready to take on your day, completely hangover-free.

There is a last little bit of maintenance we can do to make sure you feel amazing for the whole day.

Upon waking up, you'll probably want to drink a large glass of water. Grab some pink Himalayan sea salt and mix about a teaspoon in with your water.

Your adrenal glands have been stressed from all the alcohol drinking. This will alleviate much of the stress and give you a little spark of energy too.

Use that spark to go brew some coffee. While that's brewing, bust out your blender.

After the coffee is fully brewed, pour it into the blender and add 1 tablespoon of grass-fed butter for every 1 cup of coffee brewed.

Do the same thing with MCT Oil. Fire up the blender for 15 seconds, then pour your blended buttered, MCT oiled coffee into your favorite cup.

Relax and enjoy.

This butter coffee will knock out any lingering inflammation caused by all your alcohol drinking, burn off all those empty alcohol calories, clear any brain fog and give you focused energy with no late afternoon crash.

You'll be hangover-free and feel invincible.

CRACK OPEN A RECAP

Let's bullet-point the main points of this ultimate guide to hangover prevention. I want to make it absolutely simple for you to stay hangover-free without giving up your favorite booze.

- ✓ Learn how drinking alcohol affects your body
- ✓ Build a powerful pre-drinking requisite for yourself
- ✓ Boost your body's glutathione levels
- ✓ Take measures to reduce alcohol inflammation
- ✓ Stick to the clearer alcohols
- ✓ Build a powerful post-drinking requisite for yourself
- ✓ Drink water but don't over-do it
- ✓ Take activated coconut charcoal capsules before passing out
- ✓ Wake up to a glass of water with Himalayan sea salt
- ✓ Brew & blend yourself a cup of coffee with grass-fed butter and MCT oil

ONE FULL YEAR

Before we part ways...

Please try to prove what I've written in this eBook wrong. Don't assume all these hangover prevention methods work, because I say they do.

Everything in this book works for me, but it may not be the same for you. I follow what I have laid out for you here, every time I drink alcohol.

Except the part about sticking with the clear liquors, although I have been trying to implement more potato vodka over the craft beers...sometimes.

Get out there and put what I say to the test. I've surely missed a few things. And, by all means, please let me know if I have.

Do it, every weekend, for one full year. Eventually, you too, will enjoy 52 Hangover-Free Weekends!

Burn Off Your Beer Belly

Now that you've got becoming hangover-free without giving up your favorite booze nailed down, let's take all this to the next level.

If you'd like to find out more, I've put together a Free 5 Day Fat Burning Course, as part of your Free Fat Burning ToolKit - that goes into detail about how I lost 54lbs, increased my cognitive function and turned my beer belly into ripped six pack ab muscles.

Enrollment into this Free course, is officially open.

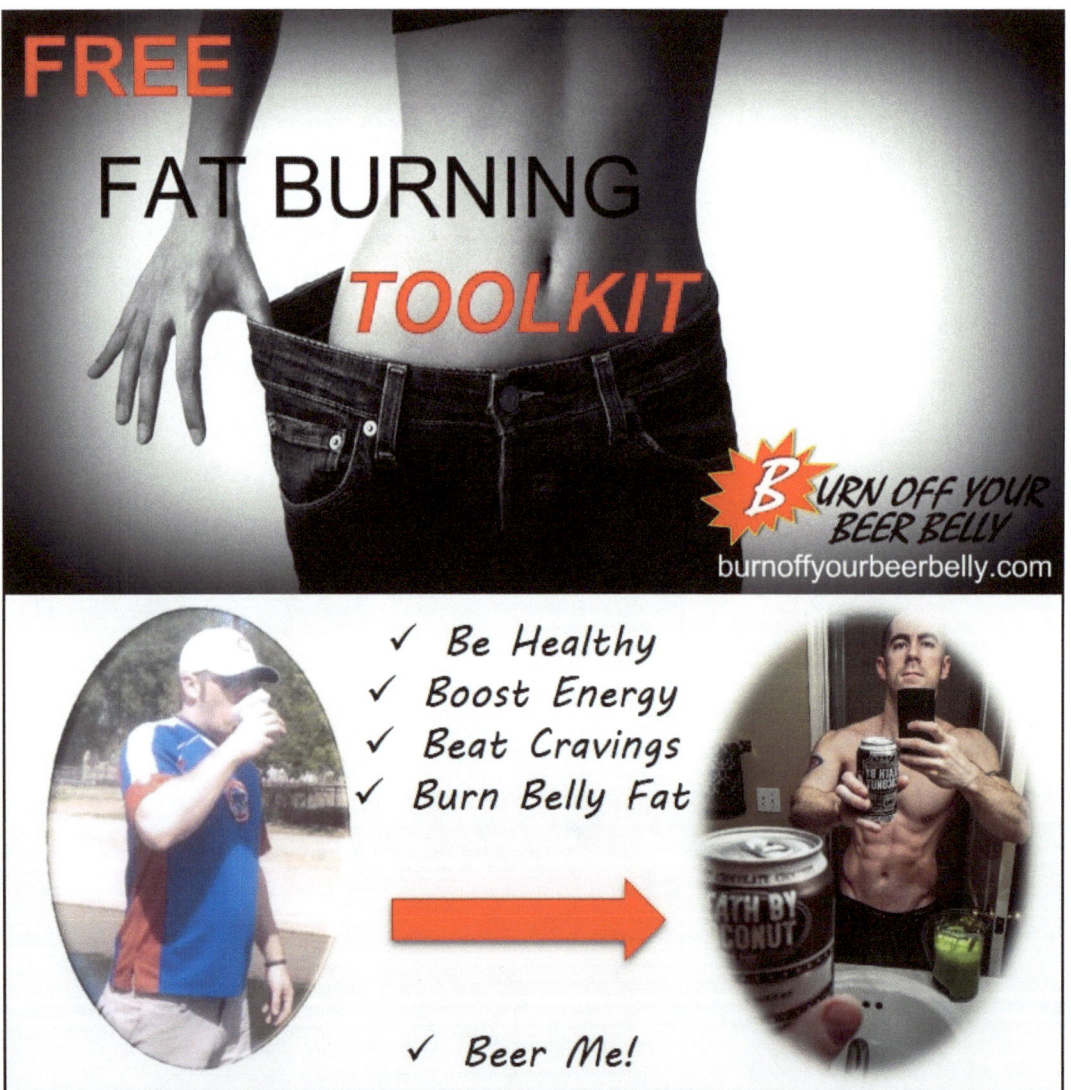

FREE FAT BURNING TOOLKIT - get all the Free tools I used to lose 54lbs, boost energy, beat cravings, prevent hangovers and burn off my beer belly:

http://www.burnoffyourbeerbelly.com/toolkit

I'll talk to you again, on the inside!

I thank you for your time and consideration.

Cheers!

Ryan Jerome
Phoenix, Arizona
2016

Did you have trouble with the formatting of this eBook?

Try downloading a PDF version of the eBook here:

52 Hangover-Free Weekends – PDF Version

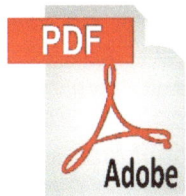

GOT QUESTIONS?

Submit a recording of your question, to be answered on the podcast, here:

http://www.burnoffyourbeerbelly.com/category/podcast/

HANGOVER QUOTES

"My first return of sense or recollection was upon waking in a strange, dismal-looking room, my head aching horridly, pains of a violent nature in every limb, and deadly sickness at the stomach. From the latter I was in some degree relieved by a very copious vomiting. Getting out of bed, I looked out of the only window in the room, but saw nothing but the backs of old houses, from which various miserable emblems of poverty were displayed . . . . At that moment I do not believe in the world there existed a more wretched creature than myself. I passed some moments in a state little short of despair . . . ."

- **William Hickey (Spenser 1913)**

"You come home, and you party. But after that, you get a hangover. Everything about that is negative."

- **Mike Tyson**

"There's nothing like taking two flights when you have a horrible hangover. It's bad when people can see actual alcohol seeping out of your disgusting pores."

- **Ike Barinholtz**

"Happiness is, waking up without a hangover."

- **Robert Black**

"I woke up hungover to the sound of my neighbor mowing the lawn. I figured he'll just have to mow around me, I'm not moving."

- **Unknown**

"Sorry you can't take a vacation because you used all your vacation days on hangovers"

- **Unknown**

"A hangover is when you open your eyes in the morning and wish you hadn't."

- **Unknown**